LAUGHTER
for the
SICK & TIRED

Sick & Tired Series:

Special Addition

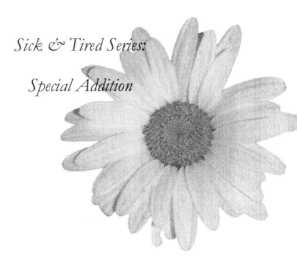

KIMBERLY RAE

Copyright © 2013 by Kimberly Rae
Cover design by Brian Thigpen
All rights reserved.
For more information on this book and the author visit
www.kimberlyrae.com.

Library of Congress Cataloging-in-Publication Data
Rae, Kimberly.
Laughter for the Sick and Tired / Kimberly Rae 2nd ed.
Sick & Tired Series, Special Addition
First Edition, June 2013
Second Edition, September 2015

All rights reserved. Non-commercial interests may reproduce portions of this book without the express written permission of the author, provided the text does not exceed 500 words. When reproducing text from this book, include the following credit line: "Laughter for the Sick and Tired by Kimberly Rae, www.kimberlyrae.com. Used by permission."

Printed in the United States of America

ISBN-13: 978-1482019520
ISBN-10: 1482019523

Sick and Tired Series

SICK & TIRED
But You Don't Look Sick!
It's Not Fair—Giving Yourself Permission to Grieve
Losing Your Identity to Sickness
How to Explain Your Illness so People Don't Think You're Faking It

YOU'RE SICK; THEY'RE NOT
Chronic Illness Changes Relationships
Why Did God Do This to My Family?
Illness and Your Love Language
Chronic Illness and Your Personality Type

WHY DOESN'T GOD FIX IT?
Bribing God
The What Ifs and If Onlys
Illness and Depression
God I'll Trust You If…

HELP FOR THE SICK & TIRED
Choosing the Right Doctor
The Love/Hate Relationship with Medication
You're the Expert on Your Body
Humiliation is Good for You

Find the latest *Sick & Tired* book at kimberlyrae.com.

TABLE OF CONTENTS

A Letter to You from the Author

Chapter 1: Sweet Pee & Other Medical Weirdness.....1

Chapter 2: Needle in the Neck................…...............9

Chapter 3: Back to the Beginning.........…..…...........17

Chapter 4: Oops..................................….…..……....25

Chapter 5: Just a Sliver....................….....…...............33

Conclusion..................................….................…..............39

About the Author

KIMBERLY RAE

A Letter to You From the Author

If you have chronic health problems like me, you know that sometimes what you need most is just a little dose of encouragement. Someone to say it stinks, you're not alone, you can make it through this day, and I'm cheering you on.

Unfortunately what we often hear instead is, "But you don't look sick!" Well, of course we don't, because on the days we do look and feel our lousiest we stay home!

That's why I want you to have this book. For those days when you can't get out and meet a friend and laugh over a cup of coffee. For the days when you feel alone, surrounded by people who don't understand. For the days when you are close to crying and wish you had something to laugh about instead.

It stinks, but you're not alone.
You can make it through this day.
I'm cheering you on!
Sincerely,
Kimberly Rae
Fellow sickie-head

Her husband had been slipping in and out of a coma for several months yet she stayed by his bedside every single day.

When he came to, he motioned for her to come nearer.

As she sat by him, he said, "You know what? You have been with me through all the bad times. When I got fired, you were there to support me. When my business fell, you were there. When we lost the house, you gave me support. When my health started failing, you were still by my side."

She just smiled and held his hand.

He then continued, saying "When I think about it now, I think you bring me bad luck."[i]

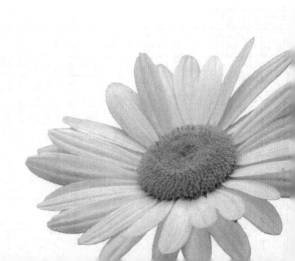

CHAPTER ONE

SWEET PEE & OTHER MEDICAL WEIRDNESS

Eat right, exercise regularly, die anyway.
Unknown

My years teaching overseas were an adventure, albeit sometimes a gross one. One day I was riding home in a rickshaw in Bangladesh and noticed a crowd standing at the fence of the medical college. They were all staring onto the college lawn.

You should know, this medical college was a frightening place to be. Broken windows. Unclean. Women paid less than two dollars to deliver babies there, but they had to bring their own bedding and materials, including someone to sleep on the floor next to their bed and cook their rice!

So it shouldn't have been all that surprising to realize that they were not particularly adept at disposing human parts that were no longer attached to humans. The crowd that day was staring at a dog. A dog and a leg. The mangy animal must have found the amputated leg in the trash bin and was dragging it around the yard. Can you imagine waking up from an amputation, looking out the window, and seeing a dog pulling your leg around? I realized that day I had been there long enough to adapt because instead of feeling ghastly, I just remember thinking, "Well, that's something I never saw before," and having the ridiculous urge to e-mail my mother about it.

≈

I sat in my Bangladeshi-style clothing and stared in slight awe at the man who was going to test my eyes for new glasses. Not that the man was awe-inspiring—I actually don't remember him at all—it was his tools. He pulled out a collection of small round lenses that he proceeded to put into framed holders perched on my nose. I'd never seen those except on *Little House on the Prairie*.

He took me into the examination room and things got even better. I sat in a chair backed against one wall of the tiny room, facing a mirror hanging only a few feet away on the opposite wall. When he started testing the different lenses, asking me to read the letters on the eye chart, I then realized the chart was actually hanging behind my head. The mirror wasn't so I could see how ridiculous I looked wearing those antique lens holders; it was there so the lens chart would be the proper distance away.

I suppose it could have been worse. The chart could have been in Bengali rather than English. As I can't read the ninety-three letters in the Bengali language, the man might have decided I was blind, and I never would have gotten a decent pair of glasses.

≈

One of the medical struggles I had in every culture I've lived in was food. Having hypoglycemia (low blood sugar), I'm not supposed to eat sweets. However, in most countries, hospitality is extremely important, and it's not polite to refuse what is offered to you. Hence my problem in Bangladesh when they'd say, "If you love me, you'll eat more," and then proceed to give me dough balls soaked in syrup. Don't tell anyone, but one day when my hostess left the room, I stuffed one of the balls into a bag in my purse.

In Uganda, they would bring us each a glass bottle of Coke® to enjoy. Sugary drinks are even worse than sugary food if you have hypoglycemia, but I was blessed one day to have come with friends who were ready to help. Ken, the only guy in the group, loved Coke, so we devised a plan. He would drink his and then when the hostess left the room, we would switch. I would hold the empty bottle and he would drink my full bottle for me. This worked great until the hostess returned, saw Ken's second empty bottle and, pleased that he enjoyed it, got him another one! It was even funnier knowing we were headed to a village with no bathroom.

≈

We may tend to think of some cultures as less advanced than ours, but sometimes I'm not so sure. In Asia, they know how to test for diabetes without anyone having to take blood, without any doctor bill, without even having to pee in a cup and give it to a stranger (which seems pretty un-advanced if you ask me).

Go pee on the ground, and if the ants come, you have diabetes. Diabetics release extra sugar in the urine, so if ants are attracted to your urine it's because there's sugar in it. Brilliant! In Indonesia, the word for diabetes is literally translated, "sweet pee."

So if you're wondering if you have diabetes but don't want the hassle of doctors and tests, you can try it yourself in your own back yard. Just make sure no one's looking first.

LAUGHTER FOR THE SICK & TIRED

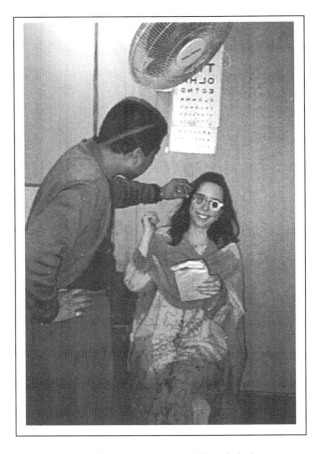

Me in the eye exam room in Bangladesh,
complete with crooked eye chart behind my head.

A good, hearty LAUGH relieves physical tension and stress, leaving your muscles relaxed for up to 45 minutes afterward.[ii]

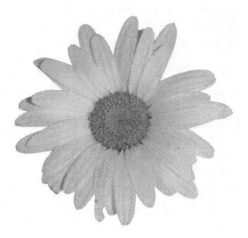

Nancy's Story:

My husband, Gary, was just diagnosed with prostate cancer. We called the insurance company to see if it would cover his treatments. We were both talking to the woman over the computer. We gave her the names and code numbers for the disease and the treatment. Then she asked, "Now which one of you would this treatment be for?"

From Real Medical Charts (supposedly):

*Patient has chest pain if she lies on her left side for over a year.

*On the second day the knee was better and on the third day it had completely disappeared.

*Patient was released to outpatient department without dressing.

*Discharge status: Alive but without permission.

*Patient has left his white blood cells at another hospital.

*She is numb from her toes down.[iii]

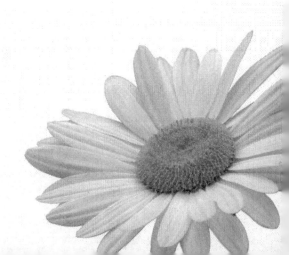

CHAPTER TWO

NEEDLE IN THE NECK

*Isn't it a bit unnerving that doctors call
what they do "practice"?
George Carlin*[iv]

My medical mishaps don't seem to come in isolated incidents. They like to cluster together and gang up on me. Like my first big hospitalization back in 2007. I had pneumonia, pleurisy, and a couple of other long words that could be fatal.

After waiting four hours in the ER waiting room, then waiting some more in the ER, I was finally assigned a room and was glad for it. Oddly, it didn't have a call button or any other amenities. I had to wander into the hallway in that totally immodest hospital gown if I needed something. We found out later it was the room for mentally unstable patients and thus the lack of small things, or big things for that matter. (Since I had lived overseas, one nurse was afraid I had the bird flu. I heard her outside my room telling another nurse, "Put your mask on. You don't know what she has!")

When they decided I was going to be staying in the hospital and thus needed a non-ER room, this caused a fiasco. They could not transfer me to a regular room because no one had officially authorized me to the mentally unstable room. So they had to do some song and dance about getting me authorized to the mental room so I could leave it. By then I was feeling a little mentally unstable, so maybe I should have stayed.

Once in my new room, I thought my troubles were over. I was wrong. Apparently this particular hospital was having trouble with its nursing staff (this story is not a complaint about nurses; nurses are awesome, just these specific ones had issues). My personal trouble with them started when one of them told me to keep track of my own urine output because I was a "bright girl" and could figure it out myself. Okay. Then my blood tests got lost and, if I heard correctly, my red juicy stuff got accidentally switched with some guy who had a liver problem. Glad they figured that out before they treated me for it!

The night nurses were wonderful and I was so thankful for them, even when they did have to stick me four times to get blood out of me. That wasn't their fault; it was my disagreeable veins.

The day shift, however, got stranger. My IV site got red and swollen, so I pushed the call button and asked for help. Waited. Pushed it again. Waited. Why didn't someone come?

I got up and trudged to the door, opening it to see several nurses hanging out and chatting in the hallway. One was ordering something from a catalog over the phone. I guess my presence got them moving because the one with the catalog came in and changed my IV, all while still ordering shoes.

A couple of days later, a wonderful doctor came in, sat down, and told me to tell him about my adrenal problem. He listened and believed me and likely saved my life, because he ordered the stress doses of cortisol my body needed. He also ordered I be sent to ICU.

Those three letters scared me. ICU. Wasn't that where people went when they were dying? In church, if a prayer request had "ICU" in it, everyone gave a little gasp, so it had to be awful, right?

The ICU was wonderful, and I have to say I got a real kick out of how the nurse there almost fell out of her chair when my husband called (he'd gone on to Indonesia because pneumonia wasn't that big of a deal and I should be out of the hospital in two days—oops) and she heard me tell about the nurse ordering shoes.

Some days later a surgeon came to visit and told me they hadn't been able to drain the infection out of my lungs with syringes (fun) and he was going to have to go in and scrape the infection from my left lung. "Do you give me permission to do this surgery?" he asked.

"What happens if I don't?"

"You die."

I laughed. "Well, I guess that narrows things down a bit!"

I did have the surgery. I did survive. And afterward because my veins were blowing and rolling so much they couldn't get anything else out of them, the surgeon came in to give me a Central IV. I'd never heard of one before, but it's a nifty little contraption where they stick you in your chest, thread a wire-like apparatus through to a major blood bank, and the part that sits "above ground" has lots of little IV ends to take blood from or give medicine to. No more sticks. This sounded like a great idea.

As he was putting it in, which was very not fun, he told me that sometimes the needle doesn't go down like it should, but rather up into the jugular. I laughed. Funny joke.

He wasn't joking. Mine did. I felt it poking my neck, ready to puncture something that should not be punctured. Obviously, this was something I wanted remedied. The surgeon told me he would fix it. Tomorrow.

Tomorrow? Are you kidding?

No, he wasn't. I think he figured since they were going to put me out for some other reason the next day, he'd just fix it then and wouldn't have to listen to my opinions on severe pain. That was a long night.

After two weeks, including nine days in ICU, I got to go home, where I faced a long recovery in bed listening to my son's *Thomas the Tank Engine* videos, which might possibly be worse than a needle in the neck when you're sick and tired and tapering off massive doses of steroids.

Since my lungs were still sore, yelling wasn't an option if I needed help, so my husband—now home thankfully—devised a plan to get his attention. He brought in a metal pot and serving spoon so I could bang the pot to call him

Good idea. Bad execution. When you're that exhausted, you don't have much energy for banging on a pot. I finally just picked up the pot and shook it, trying to get the spoon to make noise, but it was less than effective. I can't remember if we ever figured out a good system, but these days, now that we both have cell phones, I could just text him to come help me.

Unless he was on the phone already, ordering shoes or something.

LAUGHTER FOR THE SICK & TIRED

According to The British Dental Health Foundation, a smile gives the same level of stimulation as eating 2,000 chocolate bars. The results were found after scientists measured brain and heart activity in volunteers as they were shown pictures of smiling people, and given money and chocolate.[v]

(I don't really believe that. I'm all for smiling, but some things just can't compare to 2,000 bars of chocolate.)

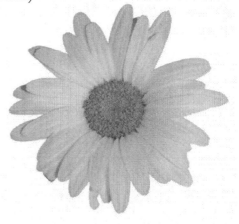

Rachel's Story:

Someone asked me about the slash/scar across my neck. I'd had my thyroid removed, but me and my talent for vocabulary told them I'd had my appendix removed. They looked at my neck funny but didn't say anything.

Appendectomy…thyroidectomy… whatever.

Iain speaks frantically into the phone, "My wife is pregnant, and her contractions are only two minutes apart."

"Is this her first child?" the doctor queries.

"No, you idiot!" Iain shouts. "This is her husband."[vi]

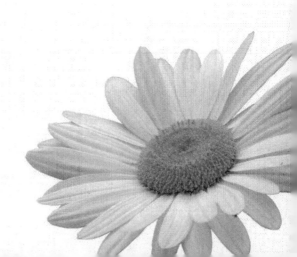

CHAPTER THREE

BACK TO THE BEGINNING

I told the doctor I broke my leg in two places.
He told me to quit going to those places.
Henry Youngman[iii]

I was nearly born in a tunnel. Perhaps that was an omen of mishaps to come when I and the medical world would meet—or rather collide.

My mother, convinced I was ready to arrive on the scene, went to the hospital only to be told to return home. False labor. Seems it wasn't very false, because as my father drove home my mom had to order him to go back. She was pretty worried I was going to come while they were driving through a long, long underwater tunnel near the hospital.

The hospital where I was born in Portsmouth, Virginia was a military hospital during the Civil War. Under the hospital was a dungeon used for Yankee prisoners. During the height of my southern mother's pain, when my northern father was apparently being less than helpful—or perhaps too helpful—she told him to "go to the dungeon with the rest of the Yankees!"

He must have forgiven her; they're still married.

≈

I had random symptoms growing up, but nothing that seemed connected. My stomach hurt as a kid, and I remember having to take these little blue pills. Once I decided to try to hide my little blue pill instead of taking it. I put it in my glass of iced tea, which shows how young I was because it didn't occur to me, until the bright blue pill was floating in the glass, that clearish-brownish liquid wasn't going to hide anything. That partially dissolved little thing was nasty to get down after that. I also recall dropping one down the floor vent once, but I'm not sure if that was a real memory or just wishful thinking.

In high school my stomach was still a wreck, but it was my normal so how was I to know? I'd get painful stomach cramps in chapel and I thought maybe it was God, trying to get me to pay attention when I was daydreaming. Now I know it wasn't God; it was just my intestines.

≈

My first real medical fiasco was when I had my wisdom teeth removed. All of them were bone impacted, which sounds pretty cool if you like that sort of thing. I was going to be given anesthesia for the first time in my life, so they sat me alone in a little room and proceeded to freak me out with a video on all the terrible things that might happen to me because they were putting me out. Like dying. Having to sign a paper that basically says if I kick off it's not their fault is not a great way to start the day.

So when it was time to put that little gas mask over my mouth and nose, at first I breathed hesitantly, not wanting to get too much of the stuff just in case it was going to kill me. However, after thinking it through, I started imagining what might happen if I didn't breathe in enough of the stuff, like waking up while they're digging my teeth out of my bone, able to feel all the pain but not communicate or move. After that I practically hyperventilated I was breathing in so hard.

Eventually I woke up minus several teeth that had never actually bothered me beforehand. I expected to get better quickly, like friends and family who had not had trouble. I of course proved to be the exception. It was horrible and took weeks to recover.

And then things got weird. I noticed little black chunks in my mouth and upon further investigation discovered they were coming from the holes in my gums where my teeth used to be. I worked at getting them out, thinking they must be tiny bits of the steak I'd eaten. Gross.

Finally, I went back to ask for help with these never-ending steak bits that I kept finding. That was when they chose to tell me that the medicated strips they had stuffed into my gums sometimes rotted on certain people rather than dissolving. Oh, and if you don't get them out, you might die. As I was leaving soon for Africa to work with orphans, planning to stay four years, that would have been an adventure, having my mouth rotting out and me still thinking it was that stubborn piece of steak!

Thanks to that little incident I learned to study up on things that doctors might neglect to tell you. You never know when there's potentially fatal stuff rotting away in your mouth, after all.

LAUGHTER FOR THE SICK & TIRED

LAUGHTER triggers the release of endorphins, the body's natural feel-good chemicals. Endorphins promote an overall sense of well-being and can even temporarily relieve pain.[viii]

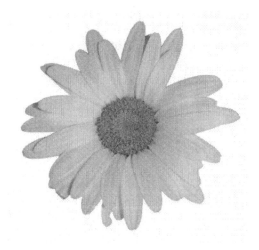

Tammy's Story:

It was my first appointment with an acupuncturist, a cute 90-poundish Chinese man who was 75. He was removing the 43 needles out of my backside when he informed me, "You probably shouldn't drink too much today as you have 43 new holes in you." He quietly laughed—"teeheeheehee."

Doctor Khan was giving a lecture to a group of medical students at the city hospital.

Pointing to the x-ray, he explained, "As you can see, this patient limps because his right fibula and tibia are radically arched."

The doctor looked up at the assembled students and asked Sidney, "Now what would you do in a case like this?"

Sidney piped up, "I suppose I would limp too."[ix]

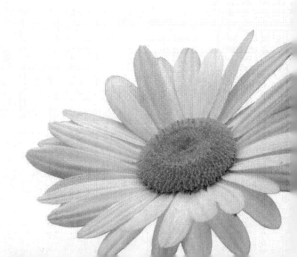

CHAPTER FOUR

OOPS

It is a mathematical fact that fifty percent of all doctors graduate in the bottom half of their class.
Unknown[x]

Just to be fair, instead of only telling you stories about when other people made not-so-helpful choices about my healthcare, I should tell you about one of the times when I was in the position of helper and completely botched things up.

I was riding home in a rickshaw on what had been a normal day of teaching children in Bangladesh. As the driver pedaled in front of me, I got to enjoy looking around at brightly painted miniature taxis, yellow bananas piled high on a motorcycle, dark water buffalo wandering down the street.

Suddenly a large truck nearby, piled high with materials and topped with people, swerved to miss a motorcycle. It tipped toward the right, swerved again, then toppled over onto its left side. I watched in horror as all the people who had been sitting on top were thrown onto the road.

Surely they were all dead.

Within seconds, people came swarming from every direction. I, too, jumped down and ran toward the accident victims.

As far as I could tell, chaos was reigning. Why was no one organizing all this? I saw a young girl, perhaps eight or nine, lying on the pavement. All my leadership skills kicked into gear. Soon I had a man carrying the girl toward a baby taxi—it would be much faster than a rickshaw. We had to get this girl to the nearest medical facility so she could be examined and helped. I was still amazed that she had lived through the ordeal in the first place.

I climbed into the baby taxi next to the girl, told the driver to take us to the nearby medical college, then tried to calm the child. She seemed to have nothing more than a few scratches, no more than had she fallen from a bicycle. It soon became obvious she feared me more than she felt the pain from the accident. I reassured her as much as I could with my very limited Bengali. I smiled and reached out to her, but she shrank away.

We rushed to the medical college. Yes, the same one where the dog was dragging the amputated leg around. When it's the only place available, you take what you can get.

The baby taxi pulled into what I guessed must be the emergency entrance. I had assumed someone from the girl's family would have arrived first and a doctor or someone capable would be waiting for the girl.

No one had arrived before us. The people at the college were looking at me in confusion. I tried to explain, but could tell quickly I was getting nowhere.

Still shaking from what I had seen, I rushed two blocks down to find my friend Debbie, who had been studying

Bengali full-time. By then I was practically begging for help. I knew I was in way over my head.

Debbie came with me back to the medical college where I was informed that the girl was no longer there. What in the world?

After a mild bit of investigating, Debbie found out that the girl's family, contrary to appearances, was more well-off than would naturally be assumed by them all riding atop a truck. As such, they had not come to the medical college for care, understandably so, but rather had chosen a private clinic.

Yet when they arrived at the clinic, their daughter was nowhere to be found.

You can imagine my humiliation. It was no wonder the poor child had been looking at me as though I had kidnapped her. For all practical purposes, I had!

As much as I dreaded it, I simply had to find the parents and apologize for making this horrible day even worse for them. I went to the private clinic and found their room, where to my chagrin I was treated like a hero. Not by the girl—she was still afraid of me—but by the mother, who gushed on and on about how wonderful I was to help her daughter.

I squirmed. I was thankful to hear that, as far as I could tell, everyone involved in the accident had lived. I only wished I had made their situation better rather than worse.

Next time I'm equally out of my element, hopefully I'll skip trying to be the hero and settle for the role of sidekick. And maybe I'll try to be a little more understanding when someone else "helps" me in a not-so-helpful way, too, in honor of the poor kid I traumatized with my good intentions.

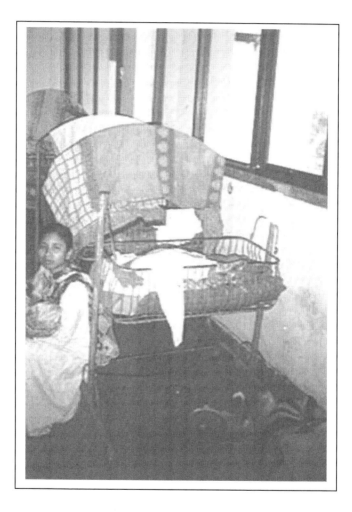

In the aforementioned medical college.
Next time you feel your medical care is sub-par,
just remember—it could be worse!

Norman Cousins, diagnosed with ankylosing spondylitis, a painful spine condition, found that a diet of comedies, like Marx Brothers films and episodes of Candid Camera, helped him feel better. He said that ten minutes of laughter allowed him two hours of pain-free sleep.[xi]

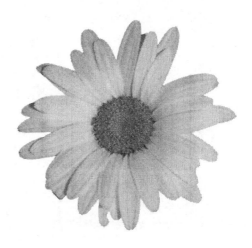

Amy's Story:

One day when I wasn't carrying my cane (for blindness), I spontaneously walked into the public library to use the computer. I sat down and picked up the log-in sheet to sign in. The librarian came over to me and whispered something. I had to ask her to repeat herself twice because neither was I wearing my hearing aids that day.

"Would you like to use the computer around the corner?"

I smiled. "Oh no, this one will be just fine."

The librarian hesitantly tapped me on the shoulder. "Umm, well, uh, that's not a computer."

Sure enough, it was a piece of typing paper—actually a sign—hanging on the wall. "In that case, I would be delighted to use the other computer," I replied. "Can you show me the way? I'm obviously blind."

I let her draw her own conclusions whether I was joking or not!

More From Real Medical Charts (supposedly):

*The baby was delivered, the cord clamped and cut and handed to the pediatrician, who breathed and cried immediately.

*The skin was moist and dry.

*She stated that she had been constipated for most of her life until 1989 when she got a divorce.

*The patient was in his usual state of good health until his airplane ran out of gas and crashed.

*The patient lives at home with his mother, father, and pet turtle, who is presently enrolled in day care three times a week.[xii]

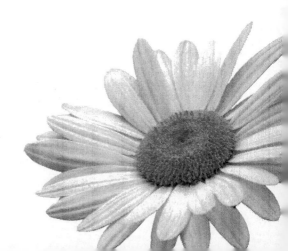

CHAPTER FIVE

JUST A SLIVER

After a lot of research, scientists have concluded that the most vitamins are found in the pharmacy.
Anonymous[xiii]

Where do we get our perspective on sickness? Does it come from environment, personality, upbringing, all of the above? I really have no idea, but if I had a choice, I would have wanted my grandpa's perspective.

Grandpa was one of my favorite people. He was brave, funny, and loved God with all his might. He was a pastor who loved people and loved to make us all laugh, though sometimes we were not laughing at his jokes so much as the fun habit he had of accidentally putting the punch line in the middle of the joke then having nothing to say once he got to the punch line part. He'd sputter a little, then start over, which of course was even funnier since we all knew what was coming.

I don't think Grandpa ever thought of himself as sick. Not after the first heart attack, or the second or third. He always would insist, "That first one wasn't really a heart attack," like it somehow made the other ones less serious if that first one wasn't legitimate. He had diabetes, and as he wasn't really supposed to eat sweets he'd say, "I'll just have a sliver," but then he'd eat two or three slivers!

Somewhere along the line he became insulin dependent, but he never made a big deal out of it so no one else did either. Sickness was just a bump in the road, something to get over and move on. Medical things were never a priority. Not even when he had to have quadruple bypass surgery on his heart. Here we all were, thinking deep and sentimental thoughts, wondering if he'd make it through the surgery. We watched as they started to wheel him away when I saw him lift his head and raise his hand to get our attention. It might be his last words. What great message would this brilliant orator leave us?

"Watch the cholesterol!" he joked, grinned, then was gone from sight.

He did make it through the surgery, and in recovery he would talk to every visitor about them, not about himself. He wanted to know if his doctors and nurses knew Jesus, if they were ready for heaven. He was ready, so why bother worrying about him and his heart? He was fine. For Grandpa, this body was just a place to hang out till it was time to go be with God, so no matter what happened to him, he was always headed toward something better, something to look forward to.

You can see why I'd love to have been gifted with his attitude about pain and sickness. It seems, however, I tend to follow more after my grandmother's way of thinking. If ever there were two opposites, it was Grandma and Grandpa. Where Grandpa would rush forward, Grandma would hold back, cautious, worried.

I wasn't always like her. Back before sickness was part of my everyday life, I would laugh at how Grandma would bring home a new prescription and sit down at the dining room table to read every possible side effect aloud. "None of that's going to happen to you," I'd say in the patronizing tone of the young and a little too self-certain.

After a few years of maturity, and several trips to urgent care with those not-gonna-happen side effects, now I'm the one reading the potential side effects out loud!

Both of them are in heaven now, totally pain and sickness free. I miss them. Though I'll probably always naturally be more like Grandma than Grandpa, perhaps I can choose the good from both sides. Maybe I can find humor despite illness, but also have compassion for those who cannot ignore their pain (like me). I'll probably always struggle with worrying about my symptoms and those possible side effects, but maybe someday I can write a funny book about them. Oh, wait, that's what I'm doing right now.

Well in that case, let me tell you about this one medication that might make me grow a beard....

LAUGHING 100 times is the equivalent to 10 minutes on a rowing machine for your cardiovascular system, or 15 minutes on an exercise bike.[xiv]

(I'd rather laugh than row any day.)

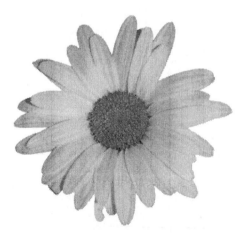

One More Story:

Barbara Johnson, in her hilarious book, *Living Somewhere Between Estrogen and Death*, tells the story of an elderly woman who went to see her daughter's gynecologist for a dreaded pap smear. While doing the exam, the doctor said, "My, aren't we fancy today!" The shocked woman left in a panic and told her daughter about the comment.

"What in the world do you think he meant by that?" she asked.

"I have no idea, Mother. What did you do to prepare for the exam?"

"Well, I showered, and I used some of that feminine deodorant spray in your bathroom," the mother replied.

The daughter paused, then said, "I don't have any feminine deodorant spray, Mother."

"Yes you do—that tall pink-and-gold can."

"Mother! That's not deodorant. That's gold-glitter hairspray!"[xv]

More Real Medical Charts (supposedly):

*Occasional, constant, infrequent headaches.

*Coming from Detroit, this man has no children.

*Patient was alert and unresponsive.

*Bleeding started in the rectal area and continued all the way to Los Angeles.

*When she fainted, her eyes rolled around the room.

*The patient was to have a bowel resection. However he took a job as a stockbroker instead.[xvi]

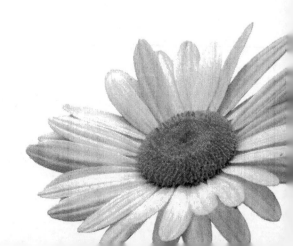

CONCLUSION

I really do take a medication that could make me grow a beard after long term use. I'm not too excited about the thought. In fact, when I told my husband, he pondered the idea for a bit, then decided, "I think I'd rather you be lethargic and clean shaven." Can't say that I blame him.

From having to have my best friend give me an emergency shot on an airplane (which was quite disconcerting to the passing stewardess) to having my blood sugar crash at the top of the Sears Tower, some days I just want to quit this whole sick thing. Unfortunately, there's no eject button for chronic illness. That fact can suck the happy right out of you if you let it.

However, there is another option than just letting illness flood our lives with negativity. The Bible says *a merry heart does good, like medicine, but a broken spirit dries the bones* (Proverbs 17:22). A bad attitude is literally bad for your body. A good attitude is good for it.

So cultivate joy. Sometimes it's hard to find, I know. Sometimes it seems to be following other people around, but when you look for it, it goes running.

For those of us with chronic illness, joy is something we have to choose. It's not going to sneak up and slap us upside the head by surprise. We're going to have to pursue it, some days relentlessly. We're going to have to grab hold and not let go.

Cultivating anything takes purposeful effort and investment. If you're cultivating a garden, you need the right soil, the right seeds, and the right nourishment. Just the same, cultivating joy needs a willing heart, some good resources, and in my opinion, God's help. The joy of the Lord is my strength (Nehemiah 8:19). It can be yours, too.

What about resources? Whatever makes you smile, or better yet, laugh, is worth investing in. I love John McPherson comics and Tim Hawkins videos (you can watch a bunch of those on You Tube for free!). Buy yourself a pretty box and fill it with things that make you smile. I have a special photo album just for my favorite funny pictures. Make your own book of comics or jokes or happy quotes. If you can't think of any funny stories of your own, grab the other books in the *Sick and Tired* series and laugh at mine!

Next time you feel like crying, instead choose joy, find something to laugh about, and see if it doesn't do you a world of good.

LAUGHTER FOR THE SICK & TIRED

KIMBERLY RAE

Want More?

Check out Kimberly Rae's book
SICK & TIRED:
Empathy, Encouragement, and Practical Help for those Suffering with Chronic Health Problems

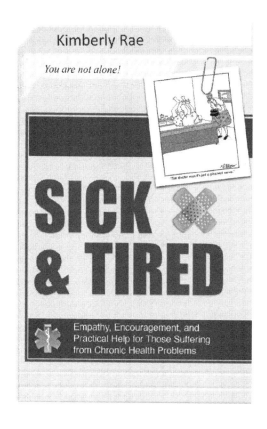

The following pages are a free excerpt. Enjoy!

Excerpt: SICK & TIRED

INTRODUCTION

Be careful about reading health books.
You may die of a misprint.
Mark Twain

Sometimes I want to slap a sticky note on my forehead that says, "I am sick. No, I don't look sick at this moment. But I am not faking having a disease just because I'm not in a wheelchair, and I am not a freak."

Now, I am aware walking around with a note like that on my head would actually put me in the freak category. Not to mention all those words would only fit on a Post-It note if I wrote it very, very small, and then people would have to get really close to me to read it, and that might just put me over the edge. I'm really into my personal space.

The thing is, I don't like talking about having chronic health problems that interfere with my life. I don't like the way people look down, over, and around me when they realize I have a chronic illness. Or worse yet, the suspicious way their eyes narrow when they decide it's all in my head, or I'm a hypochondriac.

Why does it bother me to tell people I have health problems? Doesn't everybody at some point? I suppose that's the crux right there. For most people, the difference is in the "some point" part. They have a problem. They go to the doctor. Doctor fixes it. Life moves on. It was a small, annoying inconvenience.

For me, and likely for you since you're reading this, your problem is not so temporary. You've got it for life, or until science finds a cure, which for some diseases is as likely as winning the lottery when you haven't even bought a ticket. So we make people nervous.

Nobody wants to have a condition that affects their social outings, work choices, family life, and just general day-to-day stuff. Nobody picks that for what they want to be when they grow up. "Oh teacher!" The kindergartener excitedly raises his hand. "When I grow up, I want to have a chronic illness and have people say how strong and courageous I am for enduring it even though I don't have any choice in the matter! Woo-hoo."

Instead, Americans spend billions trying to avoid anything that even smells like sickness. Our country has enough pills, vitamins, and herbal remedies to make you sick even if you started out healthy, or at least to make your urine turn neon yellow—which is an interesting phenomenon, though likely not worth all the money it took to make it happen.

We all desperately want to be well. And why not? Being well means you get to be as active as you want to be and in charge of your own daily schedule: How much sleep to get. What to eat. What job to choose, or how many children to have.

For those of us with chronic illness, we've had to give up some or all of those freedoms. And they probably didn't seem like freedoms at the time. We likely took them for granted until our bodies took them from us. Now here we are, active brains inside limited, broken bodies. But as technology has yet to create a way to get an entire body transplant, we're stuck with it.

Unless, of course, you have a neurological problem, as I think I might, in which case I'm sorry about your brain. Getting a brain transplant is a seriously bad idea. You would not even know who you were, and would not appreciate how much better you were feeling.

I would like to trade in my health problems and be well again. I sometimes think that would be getting my life back. But the truth is, this is my life, and as I have come to (almost) accept that fact and make the best of it, I think there's hope for me.

Maybe not to cease being a freak to some, but to cease seeing myself as a victim, as a traumatic case, or even as a lesser being because of my illness.

That being the goal, maybe I'll remove the hypothetical Post-It note from my forehead and put it in my back pocket, to be removed periodically and waved in people's faces only when I'm having a tough day.

It's a start anyway.

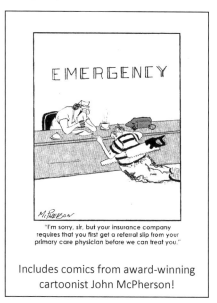

Includes comics from award-winning cartoonist John McPherson!

Also in the *Sick & Tired* Series:

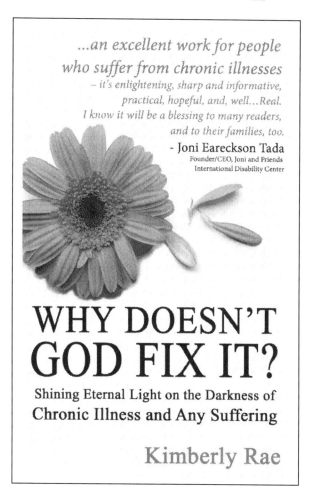

Bribing God
The If Onlys and What Ifs
Illness and Depression
When the Mountain Won't Move

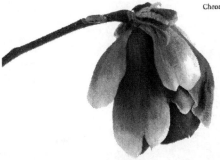

YOU'RE SICK THEY'RE NOT

Relationship Help for People with Chronic Illness And Those Who Love Them

...an amazing read for both my husband and myself and helped us to focus on us and not just my illness.
- Jennifer
Chronic Illness Sufferer

Kimberly Rae

How Different Personalities Respond to Stress
Love Languages and Chronic Illness
How to Avoid Friction over the Holidays
What to do about the People Who Just Don't Get It

Coming 2016

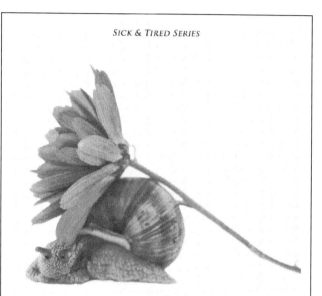

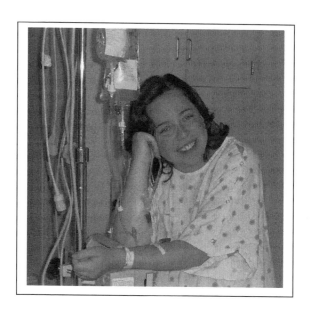

ABOUT THE AUTHOR

Kimberly Rae lived in Bangladesh, Uganda, Kosovo and Indonesia before Addison's disease brought her permanently back to the US. Rae has been published over 350 times and has work in 5 languages. Her Christian suspense/romance novels on international human trafficking (*Stolen Woman, Stolen Child,* and *Stolen Future*) are all Amazon bestsellers.

Rae now lives in the foothills of the Blue Ridge Mountains in North Carolina with her husband and two children.

Find out more or contact the author at
www.kimberlyrae.com.

Bibliography

[i] http://www.most-funny-jokes.com/funny-medical-jokes-by-my-side.html
[ii] http://www.helpguide.org/life/humor_laughter_health.htm
[iii] *http://www.medi-smart.com*
[iv] http://coolfunnyquotes.com
[v] http://www.helpguide.org/life/humor_laughter_health.htm
[vi] *http://www.guy-sports.com/humor/jokes/jokes_doctor.htm*
[vii] http://coolfunnyquotes.com
[viii] http://www.helpguide.org/life/humor_laughter_health.htm
[ix] *http://www.guy-sports.com/humor/jokes/jokes_doctor.htm*
[x] http://www.buzzle.com/articles/funny-get-well-sayings.html
[xi] Anatomy of An Illness, http://www.webmd.com/balance/features/give-your-body-boost-with-laughter
[xii] http://www.most-funny-jokes.com/funny-medical-jokes-actual-medical-charts.html
[xiii] http://coolfunnyquotes.com
[xiv] http://www1.villanova.edu/content/dam/villanova/studentlife/documents/healthcenter/Health%20Center/stress_less_laugh_more.pdf
[xv] Living Somewhere Between Estrogen and Death, by Barbara Johnson, 1997, Thomas Nelson Inc. Used with permission.
[xvi] http://www.most-funny-jokes.com/funny-medical-jokes-actual-medical-charts.html

Made in the USA
Middletown, DE
14 June 2018